# Contents

# Introduction - You're Not Alone

Before we even get started, there are a few important things that need to be stated. Losing weight is a mind game. If you change your mind, you'll change your body. It's inevitable.

When we say "change your mind", it doesn't mean changing your mind from eating cookies to gobbling cake.

What we're talking about here is the mindset behind all weight loss. It doesn't matter what your age or sex is... the principles are the same.

First, you need to stop hating your body. Way too many women have negative images of themselves. They feel that they're fat and ugly while all the other women are better.

You may have coveted the 'thigh gap' but can't even find clothes your size at The Gap.

***"Why can't I look like her?"*** *...* ***"It sucks being me!"*** *...* ***"I have horrible fatty genes!"***

These are just some of the ways women beat themselves up. Here's the truth...You need to love yourself for what you are... flab, rolls, cellulite and all.

You need to start this weight loss journey from a place of self-love.

If you don't change this mindset, even when you lose the weight, you will still have negative self-image issues. You will never be good enough for you.

Accept yourself... and from there you can improve. This is a journey and not an overnight miracle.

**Look in the mirror. That's your competition**. Not anyone else.

You also need to understand that you CAN lose weight. By assuming that you have 'fat genes' or that it's more difficult for you to lose weight, you make it a self-fulfilling prophecy.

There will be times when you slip up. This is inevitable and par for the course. When pursuing any worthy goal, the journey is never linear.

It's often fraught with little setbacks, slip ups, mistakes, etc. What you need to understand is that every setback is a set up for a comeback.

During those times when you slip up on your diet, don't throw in the towel and give up just because you made one mistake in your diet.

If you eat a slice of cake after work, don't blame yourself and go crazy the rest of the day by eating whatever else comes your way. Acknowledge your mistake and strive not to make any more.

If you are on track for the next few days, this one small slip up will be negligible. If you throw your diet out of the window and give up, you can rest assured that the weight will pile back on.

You are not your mistake. Acknowledge, correct it, and avoid future mistakes and KEEP MOVING FORWARD. That is the only way to succeed.

You're definitely in control of your body and can change for the better if you know what to... and this book will tell you what to do.

All that you need to do is follow it to the letter and you will reach your desired weight. In the process, you will gain energy, become stronger, feel happier and have a sense of accomplishment that just can't be described.

Does that excite you? It should!

Read on.

# Chapter 1 - The Struggle Is Real

Yes, it is.

This is what the weight loss companies and diet pills manufacturers don't want you to know. Weight loss is a difficult process.

The concept is brain dead simple. All you need to do is burn more calories than you consume. That's all it is. If you remove all the fluff and hype, it always boils down to this one principle.

You need to eat the right foods in the right quantities and get sufficient exercise.

The diet pill companies will tell you that you can achieve staggering results – ***"Lose 12 Pounds in 7 Days!"*** without starving yourself. Easy weight loss! That's always their angle.

Common sense will tell you that these pills will never work. After all, how can you lose weight by eating something else?

To convince you that these pills work, the supplement companies will list a whole range of ingredients that sound exotic and supposedly have fat burning properties.

Women believe this hype because the truth is a bitter pill to swallow. Cleaning up your diet and exercising is difficult. Taking weight loss pills is easy.

And everybody wants easy.

Easy often leads to disappointment, regret, a loss of time and money. This is a heavy price to pay because most often, you'll never see any results.

That's why you see women going from pill to pill. That's why new weight loss supplements keep hitting the market. When people realize that it's not working, they try the next product and the next and the next... This vicious cycle just doesn't end.

You need to understand that in most cases, you gained the weight gradually. Nobody wakes up 20 pounds heavier overnight. Your body got fatter over time.

In order to lose the fat, it will take time. This book says that you'll transform your body in 28 days… and it will. If you do what it says.

It doesn't make wild promises of losing 20 pounds in a week. In best case scenarios, you might lose 3 to 4 pounds a week. In 4 weeks, you'll lose about 12 pounds… or maybe 8.

It all depends on your body. The more excess weight you have, the more weight you'll lose. It's a strange contradiction but generally, fatter people lose weight faster.

The leaner you get, the more challenging it becomes.

Whatever the case may be, 28 days is a good time frame to aim for. You will definitely see the difference

There is a quote in the fitness industry.

**It takes 4 weeks for you to see your body changing.**

**It takes 8 weeks for your friends and family.**

**It takes 12 weeks for the rest of the world.**

**KEEP GOING**

This is very true. In 28 days, the transformation that you see will give you the motivation to keep going because you know that what you're doing works.

Most people give up because they can't see results fast enough. Usually, they've just not given themselves enough time.

You'll need to plan your weight loss and then you'll realize just how long it will take you to reach your goal. We'll be looking at this in the next chapter.

What's really important is that it keeps things realistic for you. If you're looking at an 8 week stretch to reach your dream body, you'll not lose motivation and give up after 2 weeks because you have six more weeks to go.

You also will not believe the hype that the infomercials and supplements throw at you.

You body works at its own pace. It's not affected by hype or fantasies. Weight loss is based on natural laws. You wear what you eat. You need to move more... and you need to stay the course. This is what transforms your body.

It doesn't sound glamorous or fun... but the truth seldom does.

Nevertheless, you can lose weight. You ALWAYS can. Now let's move on to the next chapter where I show you just how long it'll take you to reach your desired weight.

# Chapter 2 - Planning & Tracking Your Progress

The first thing you need to do is to check what your daily caloric deficit should be.

Being at a daily caloric deficit is the most important factor that determines if you will succeed or fail.

You could eat clean, watch your diet and exercise daily... BUT... if you're at a caloric surplus, you will never see your weight drop.

This is the reason why so many people struggle to lose weight and never see progress.

So, what is a caloric deficit?

It simply means a shortage in the amount of calories consumed relative to the amount of calories required for maintenance of current body weight.

In other words, you're consuming fewer calories than your body uses. Now your body has no choice but to tap into its fat stores for fuel.

This is the only way you will deplete your body's fat stores and lose weight.

Ideally, you should aim for around a 500-calorie deficit daily.

You don't need to obsess over the numbers and aim for perfection. As long as you're within the 400 to 600 range, you'll be just fine and lose weight steadily.

You'll now be shown 3 different numbers.

**Maintenance** means that if you consume this number of calories, your weight will neither go up nor go down.

**Fat loss** denotes a caloric deficit. This is the number that you need to aim for in order to lose weight.

**Extreme Fat Loss** is an indicator that you should not drop your calories below this number.

So, if you wish to lose 20 pounds and you're losing about 2 pounds a week, you'll be looking at a time frame of 10 weeks... that is about 2 and a half months.

It seems long, doesn't it?

Here's what Earl Nightingale once said – *"Don't let the fear of the time it will take to accomplish something stand in the way of your doing it. The time will pass anyway; we might just as well put that passing time to the best possible use."*

Even if it takes you 10 weeks, go for it.

While this guides states 28 days, these 28 days are for you to see a transformation. To actually see results!

Most women never see any results. This guide gives you results... However, if you need 10 weeks, you're not going to achieve it in 28 days. If we follow the example mentioned above, you'll lose 8 pounds in 28 days.

It may not seem like much, but it is definitely going to be a visible difference. Your face will become slimmer. Your belly and thighs may shrink a little. You'll be amazed.

And that's the whole point of this book... To show you what's possible... and from there you keep going. If it takes you ten weeks, you just keep doing what you've been doing these 28 days till you reach the ten weeks.

You must stay the course!

Success is nothing more than a few simple disciplines, practiced every day.

What gets measured gets managed. So, it's imperative that you measure your progress and keep a close eye on your diet and training.

The first thing you'll need to do is weigh yourself on a weighing scale. You should do this once a week on the same day and at the same time.

Do not weigh yourself daily because your weight will fluctuate and it can be demoralizing. Once a week will do and it will reflect any weight loss.

Do note that the scale weight only gives you a general idea but it is not indicative of body composition.

For example, if you lost 3 pounds of fat and gained 2 pounds of muscle, the scale will only show a loss of 1 measly pound. This can be very misleading. You'd actually have made good progress and will look different since fat takes up a lot more space than muscle.

That is why you also need to take photos of your body once every 2 weeks. With photos, the difference in your appearance will be more evident and you'll feel more motivated.

Many people are much more amazed to see before and after photos instead of just a difference in numbers on a scale.

If possible, get your bodyfat percentage measured. You can ask your doctor to do this and he or she will probably use calipers to determine your bodyfat percentage.

This is an accurate measurement to go by and your goal will be to lower your bodyfat percentage to what's ideal for you.

Using a tape measure to record down the measurements of different parts of your body is helpful too. You can encircle the tape around the middle of your thigh, your arm, hips, chest, etc.

It's important that you measure the same places in future to keep things accurate. With time, you'll notice the inches dropping. Even if the scales show no difference after 2 weeks of exercise, the tape measure will definitely show you if you have become smaller.

Muscle is a lot denser than fat and takes up much less space.

In the first 3 to 4 weeks, it may seem like the results are slow. Losing a few pounds here and there may make it all seem like a total waste of time. You must understand that there are changes happening in you.

The body is adapting. Your metabolic rate is increasing. The body is starting to tap into its fat stores for fuel.

All this is happening on the inside but you do not see obvious results on the outside. This discourages the majority of women who quit on their weight loss program within the first month. Most give up after 2 weeks!

The take a break and go back to their poor eating habits and sedentary lifestyle. 2 months later they decide to lose weight again. When does it ever end?

This is the biggest mistake. You've just turned on the ignition and before the pedal hits the metal, you've given up.

Motivation is what gets you started. Habit is what keeps you going.

When you embark on a weight loss journey, give yourself an end date 90 days later. Do not stop before you reach that 90 days or you reach your weight loss goal.

There may be occasions where you slip-up on your diet. There may be times when you skip your workouts. There may even be weeks where there is no change in weight. Despite all these, keep going till you reach the 90-day mark.

If you hate starting over, stop giving up. Three months from now, you will thank yourself. Do not give up on yourself and kill off your weight loss dreams before they have time to bloom.

Most visible weight loss can be seen after 90 days. That's about 3 months. You absolutely must give yourself 3 months.

Track your progress weekly and if things don't seem to be changing for the better, tweak your workouts and diet.

This is the best way to lose weight without losing your way.

# Chapter 3 - Mastering Hunger & Conquering Emotional Overeating

Let's face it. If you want to lose weight, you're going to have to eat less. Yes... yes... You don't want to. You enjoy eating. Do you really have to cut down your calorie intake?

Yes.

What if you eat the same amount and just exercise? No. You still need to eat less.

Ok... ok. You'll eat the same amount, exercise like crazy and pop a few slimming pills too. That ok? No. You'll still have to eat less.

Now that we have established that fact, we can move on. When we say eat less, it doesn't mean that you will have to eat like a bird. You'll always have enough food to eat, to stay strong, fit and healthy.

The problem society faces these days is that people eat too much. They eat when they're happy. They eat when they're sad.

They eat when they're hungry and they eat when they're not hungry... out of fear that they might get hungry later.

Once you aim to cut your calories, you will definitely end up eating less than you're accustomed to. Since you're already in the habit of eating a certain quantity of food daily, the body is going to feel a little hungry.

This is normal. You're not starving. Your body needs time to adjust to the fewer calories. There will be slight discomfort and you may find yourself thinking of food often. You will need to exercise will-power and not eat. Maintaining the caloric deficit is imperative to losing the pounds.

Look at it as a challenge that you can surmount. Many women look at controlling their diet as a huge pain in the butt.

There are 7 tips in this chapter to curb your appetite. These will help to a certain extent at controlling your cravings. Do note that within a week of maintaining a caloric deficit, your appetite will naturally diminish.

The less you eat, the less you'll want to eat. You stomach will shrink and you'll require less food to feel satiated.

That may take a week or two to happen. Depending on how much you've been eating daily, it may take longer but rest assured that you will need less food as you go along.

## 7 Tips to Curbing Hunger

1. Skip breakfast.

This runs contrary to everything you've heard so far. However, studies have shown that the later in the day you have your first meal, the less you'll eat throughout the day. If you really must have breakfast, go ahead, but keep it light and make sure it is protein based. Skip the sugary cereals and white bread.

2. Drink lots of water.

It'll make you feel full and very often people mistake thirst for hunger. You also need to be sufficiently hydrated to accelerate fat loss.

3. Consume a tablespoon or 2 of virgin coconut oil daily.

It has been shown to reduce one's appetite, make a person leaner and also less prone to storing fat.

4. Stay active throughout the day.

Sedentary activities such as vegetating in front of the TV for hours, playing video games non-stop, watching movies at the cinema, etc. will automatically make you want to pop something in your mouth to munch. Avoid these activities.

## 5. Eat lots of vegetables.

Vegetables such as broccoli, spinach, carrots, cauliflower, kale, celery, etc. contain a ton of beneficial properties. Not only are they good for your health but they will also leave you feeling fuller for longer.

## 6. Use smaller plates.

This is a psychological trick. Smaller plates look fuller with less food. So, your brain automatically assumes you're eating a lot when you're not.

## 7. Go to bed earlier.

A bad habit that many people engage in is binge eating at night. This is usually because they're awake watching TV and end up feeling hungry. If you find that you're getting hungry at night, go to bed earlier. You will not struggle against cravings.

Follow the tips above and you will reduce the amount that you eat. Once you achieve this feat, your weight loss will go from being a possibility to a probability and finally, a reality. Your diet is that important to your success. Never forget that.

# Chapter 4 - Do You Need To Diet?

You don't need to diet... but you need to follow a diet.

Does that sound confusing?

Many women make the mistake of starving themselves in the hope of losing weight fast. This is counterproductive and actually works against them.

You need to be on a diet that is right for you... and most importantly, you need to be at a caloric deficit.

As long as you're at a caloric deficit, you will lose weight.

You're probably wondering... ***"What if I ate junk food and still maintained a caloric deficit?"***

In theory, yes. It's not so simple... but yes. You can lose weight even while eating fast food, processed food, and junk food... whatever they may call it. You know what these foods are.

As was mentioned in chapter 1, if you consume lesser calories than your maintenance level, you will lose weight.

Therefore, theoretically speaking, even if you were on a junk food diet the entire day but you were consuming about 500 calories lesser than your maintenance level, you will lose weight.

Many overweight or obese women, almost always have a very poor diet. It is extremely difficult for them to switch from a diet that is so high in processed/junk food to one that is clean and wholesome.

Expecting to switch your diets overnight is just setting yourself up for failure. You absolutely must do this slowly and progressively. Therefore, your best course of action will be to carry on eating the way you have, but aim for a caloric deficit.

That essentially means that you'll be consuming less junk food than you were used to. This in itself will help you lose weight.

However, since the goal is to lose weight and get healthy, your end goal should be to eliminate junk food from your diet and eat clean.

Every week, make one small positive change to your diet. If you usually have 2 cheeseburgers for lunch followed by a soda, you may replace that with a crunchy tuna wrap and a glass of cold coconut water.

Psychologically, this is easier. It's just one meal. Keep at it till this becomes a habit and you slowly but surely, replace all the junk meals with wholesome yet tasty meals.

Healthy meals can be delicious too. You are not sacrificing taste or pleasure by eating healthily. It's just a matter of getting your taste buds and body to enjoy eating healthy foods. Over time this can be achieved.

In the meantime, you may eat junk foods and still lose weight while on a caloric deficit.

You should also note that junk foods are nutrient deficient. That means, you could be eating junk food and after a short while still feel hungry. That's because your body hasn't got all the nutrients it needs. This is one reason why if your diet is poor, you always feel hungry no matter what you eat.

Also note that, there are certain processes within the body that will prevent you from losing weight beyond a certain point. The body is a highly complex organism. It will lose weight for a while since you are on a caloric deficit. However, with time, you will find it increasingly difficult to do so.

It's not merely a mathematical equation where calories in must be less than calories out. There are other factors such as the quality of the calories consumed, the thermogenic effect of the food eaten, etc.

So, ideally, you may consume junk food at a caloric deficit and over a period of a month or two, slowly wean yourself off these unhealthy foods and get on a healthy diet.

Of course, you may indulge in junk food once in a while. However, many people who have made the switch never feel the urge to eat junk food again.

One of the best ways of eating to lose weight will be to consume foods that help with the fat burning process.

By including these foods in your diet, you'll not only feel more satiated but the body will burn more calories too. Unlike weight loss supplements, these foods actually work... and they're cheaper.

**Foods That Burn Fat**

- Almomds

- Oatmeal

- Eggs

- Legumes & Beans

- Berries

- Olive oil

- Green vegetables

- Lean meats & oily fish

- Green tea

- Avocadoes

- All natural peanut butter

Just by consuming these foods, you'll be able to curb your hunger and also hasten the fat burning process.

So... while you do not need to follow a highly restricted diet and starve yourself, you should aim to consume foods that are beneficial to your health.

You'll be amazed at just how much good food you can eat when it's not processed. In the next chapter, we'll look at what the best foods are for you and what is the single best thing you can do to lose weight.

# Chapter 5 - Whole Foods and Wrong Foods

Before telling you what the good foods to eat are, here is one of the BEST ways to lose weight fast.

You ready?

## Cut Your Carbohydrate Intake and Processed Foods!

Carbohydrate intake is one of the biggest factors affecting the speed at which you lose weight. In fact, the main reason most women gain weight is because they consume too much processed carbs.

When you eat processed carbs such as donuts, pasta, white bread, white potatoes, etc. the calories quickly add up and the body has a lot of fuel.

It shuttles all the excess fuel into its fat stores and that's how you gain weight. Furthermore, the processed carbs usually cause a spike in insulin levels which indirectly lead to weight gain. A double whammy.

There is no denying that a restricted carb intake will do wonders for your fat loss. In fact, studies have shown that restricting your carbs is more effective than restricting your calories.

So, if you are on a 500 calorie deficit daily, and your carb intake is minimal, you will lose much more weight in the same span of time than you would by consuming carbs while on a deficit.

Does that make sense? In simple words, less carbs equals more fat loss. Sounds good? You bet!

When you cut down your carb intake, your body will burn more fat from its fat stores because it doesn't have much carbs to burn for fuel. So, fat loss is accelerated.

Your body's blood sugar level will drop and people suffering from diabetes will see an improvement in their condition. A restrictive carb diet also keeps type 2 diabetes at bay since your body's insulin sensitivity is on point.

Your good cholesterol levels will go up and your bad cholesterol levels will drop. Many people assume that cholesterol is linked to fat intake.

The truth is that a high carb intake also has an adverse impact on your cholesterol levels. This runs contrary to popular belief yet studies show that a low-carb diet has more positive effects on your triglycerides than a low-fat diet.

Now, it is important to note that **you should never take things to extremes**. This applies to carb restriction too.

There are diets such as the Atkins diet which is based on severe restriction of carbs for long periods of time. This is detrimental to your body because you will end up fatigued, moody and weak.

The diet is not sustainable and once you come off it, you will gain whatever weight you lost and a bit more.

Excessive carb restriction will compromise your immune system, lead to muscle loss, slow down your fat burning and put you in a weight loss plateau.

Your body's testosterone production will fall and you will have a suppressed thyroid output. You'll also develop leptin resistance which doesn't bode well for fat loss.

So, what do you do? How do you strike the right balance? You want the best of both worlds, don't you?

The only way to achieve this is with a technique that is known as carb cycling. You will avoid carbohydrates for 3 to 6 days at a time.

If you are overweight or obese and have a slower metabolism, you should aim for 5 to 6 days of minimal or zero carbs.

If you just have a few extra pounds to lose, you just need to go for 3 to 4 days with low or no carbs.

After the period of carb restriction, you will follow it with one day of carb intake. This is known as your "re-feed" day.

Consume sufficient carbs on this day and you will give your body the fuel that it needs. Your metabolism will get a boost and your body will get a surge of energy as its fuel stores get replenished.

Stick to healthy carbs such as sweet potatoes, whole grain breads, whole grain pastas, etc. You should aim for a 500 to 700 calorie surplus over maintenance level. This will put your body back in fat burning mode.

Use this technique repeatedly to accelerate your fat loss and improve your health. The day will come when you won't crave for carbs or processed junk foods.

When your body becomes healthy, its tastes will change. That's why fit people are constantly able to make wise food choices. Once you have gotten over the hump of ditching these foods, the rest is easy.

Your insulin sensitivity will improve, the pounds will drop and you will look and feel like a brand new you.

There is a saying – "Your abs are made in the kitchen, not the gym." What that means is that almost 80% of your success at weight loss or getting lean is dependent on your diet.

When it comes to weight loss, the majority of your attention must be given to your diet.

The 7 foods listed below will sabotage your weight loss efforts. There is absolutely no doubt that you have everything to gain and nothing to lose by giving these foods a pass.

The problem is that many people love these comfort foods and hate giving them up. Sugar is addictive.

The more sugary foods you eat, the more you'll crave. So, by eliminating them slowly, you'll slowly condition your body to crave for these foods less and less.

## 7 Foods You Should AVOID at All Costs!

- Doughnuts are probably one of the unhealthiest foods on the planet. They consist of nothing more than refined carbohydrates and sugar.

  They are high in calories, fats, carbs and other preservatives. Continued consumption of doughnuts will lead to weight gain digestive problems.

- Fast food. Enough said.

- Chips are just about everybody's guilty pleasure. Ah... the joys of crunching on them while watching a movie. Chips have high levels of trans fats due to the hydrogenated vegetable oils that are used to fry the chips. This will lead to weight gain and cardiovascular disease.

- French fries. It has been said that French fries are more deadly than cigarettes. There may be some truth in this.

High in trans fats and carcinogens, these foods can cause cancer.

- Bagels are another crowd pleaser. It has a very high glycemic index. It causes insulin spikes this creates inflammation in the body along with other health issues. Acne, body aches, clogged arteries, mood swings, etc. are all side effects of unstable insulin levels... and of course, weight gain.

Skip the morning bagel. It's better to skip the bagel than go for a 30 minute walk. That roughly gives you an idea of how detrimental it is.

- Microwaved popcorn. All the rage these days. Convenient, tasty and fun. Yet, they contain carcinogens and diacetyl. Both cause cancer.

- Cereals are another fat gain culprit. Most cereals are not good for your body despite being marketed as "healthy natural foods". There is hardly anything natural about cereals. They are genetically modified foods that can harm you in the long run.

Just avoiding the unhealthy foods is half the battle won. Always remember the long term effects. Don't give in to sinful pleasures in the short term which may lead to suffering in the long run.

## Proteins

Protein requires more energy to digest than carbs or fats. That means if you eat a slice of beef that's about 200 calories, hypothetically you might burn 40 calories digesting it. Whereas, eating an ice-cream will require very few calories to digest it.

That means you should be getting quite a bit of your daily calories from protein foods. Meats and legumes are awesome sources of protein. The protein will also help you gain muscle if you are on a weight training program. Aim for about 0.8 grams per pound of bodyweight.

The protein will build more muscle. When you have more muscle, you end up burning more fat. This is a good cycle to be in. That is why you may notice that people who are muscular and fit get away with eating more. Their muscles are burning more calories round the clock.

Good sources of protein are skinless chicken, lean beef, tuna, sardines, chickpeas, eggs and salmon. The fish contain Omega-3 fatty acids. That makes them even more beneficial to the body.

The chemical properties in certain foods trigger off certain processes in the body that cause fat loss. So, eating these foods will make your body wake up and burn more fat.

## Green Tea

Green tea is one of them. Do not use sugar. It may not taste great but it works.

## Other Foods

Chilies, lemons, oranges, mangoes, garlic, ginger and onions are all food that contains many powerful antioxidants and nutrients that strengthen your immune system. When you are strong, your workouts will be better and you will burn more fat.

One common problem most women face when they first embark on a weight loss program is that they constantly feel hungry.

Food is always on their mind and it takes a toll on their willpower.

One way to prevent this is to consume foods that are high in fiber and digest slowly. You will feel fuller for a longer period of time.

Foods that are high in fiber are quickly digested and passed through the digestive track sooner. That means fewer calories are absorbed resulting in less tendency to gain weight.

Consume foods like oatmeal, oats, brown rice, whole grain bread and broccoli. Broccoli is so good for your body that you should make it a staple in your diet.

The goal here is to consume whole foods and not processed foods. Generally, the whole foods are found on the perimeter of most supermarkets.

As long as you avoid the food in the inner aisles and shelves, you'll be distancing yourself from the processed foods.

Last but not least, as beneficial as these foods are, they will only help you lose weight if you're on a caloric deficit and have a proper exercise regimen.

The 2 key components to any fat loss is a caloric deficit while on a balanced diet and a good exercise program. Everything else is just gravy.

So, no matter how good and clean your diet is, make sure you're still at a daily caloric deficit.

# Chapter 6 - Water Not Wine

While there is nothing wrong in drinking the occasional glass of wine, when you're trying to lose weight, almost all the fluid you consume should only be water.

The easiest way to get fat is to drink your calories. Avoid sodas, commercially sold fruit juices, sports drinks, etc. You only need water!

And you should drink lots of it.

This is why you should drink water...

- Drinking ice cold water in the morning speeds up your metabolism

- It reduces your appetite. Any time you feel like snacking, drink a glass or two of water and you'll feel full and be less likely to snack.

- It keeps you hydrated and healthy.

- Your body needs water to metabolize fat. It's part of the fat burning process.

- You'll be less likely to get dehydrated during exercise if you drink water regularly.

There's really no need to emphasize this any further. Drink enough water daily.

# Chapter 7 - The Power of Protein

This is one of the most powerful techniques to speed up weight loss.

The more proteins you consume, the faster you'll lose weight. The body uses up more calories to digest protein. Unlike fats and carbs which are quickly and easily digested, proteins burn more calories.

Never consume a carb without a protein. Never consume a fat without a protein.

Just by having the protein together with these foods, you'll prevent an insulin spike.

One of the best ways to get protein in your diet is to eat eggs.

Eggs are one of the most nutritious foods on the planet. They have received a bad rep about high cholesterol and a lot of other false information.

This is highly ironic since cereals which are detrimental to one's health are believed to be healthy, yet eggs which are truly beneficial are demonized.

This book will set the record straight. Eggs are a wonderful source of protein, omega-3 fatty acids and a lot of other beneficial nutrients.

Cholesterol in the body is due to saturated fat and trans fat and not dietary cholesterol. That means that despite what you have been told, eating the eggs with the yolk is just fine.

In fact, it's healthier since most of the nutrients are found in the yolk.

Not only are eggs a fantastic source of lean protein and heart-healthy omega-3 fatty acids, but they contain some pretty important nutrients.

Eggs are also considered to be the perfect food. They contain vitamin D, 7 grams of protein, vitamins B6, B12, choline, leucine, L-arginine and folate. You may not be familiar with what most of these vitamins are but what really matters is that they are what your body truly needs.

What truly matters is how you prepare the eggs and that you consume them in moderation. Do not fry eggs in saturated fat or in vegetable oils. Use coconut oil or olive oil. Fry them lightly or half-boil them.

The point to note is that when you are losing weight, you should mix 2 egg yolks and the rest should be egg whites. This is assuming that you're having more than 2 eggs.

The reason for this is that egg yolks though high in protein, are calorie dense. So, you want the benefits that eggs provide but you do not want to add too many calories to your diet.

If you're still on the fence about this, Rochester Centre for Obesity in America, conducted research that proved eating eggs for breakfast could limit daily calorie consumption by more than 400 calories. Isn't that fantastic?

One point to note is that if you are consuming eggs daily, you will be getting more than enough protein. It would be ideal to avoid protein shakes and other commercial protein products sold in your health stores. Ideally, we should be getting our proteins from natural sources.

Also, try and get eggs that are organic. They will contain less omega-6 fats and more omega-3 fats.

**If you're a vegetarian and don't eat eggs...**

There are many vegetables that are high in protein too. You can eat those and achieve the same benefits.

## 20 High Protein Veggies

- Peas (Green)

- Mange Tout (Edible-Podded Peas, cooked)

- Sweet Corn (Yellow)

- Succotash (Corn And Limas, cooked)

- Sprouted Beans, Peas & Lentils (Soybean Sprouts)

- Lima Beans (Cooked)

- Kale

- Broccoli Raab (Cime di Rapa, cooked)

- Parsley

- Artichokes (Globe or French)

- Spinach (Cooked)

- Mushrooms (White, cooked)

- Collard Greens

- Mustard Greens

- Broccoli

- Baby Zucchini (Courgettes)

- Garden Cress

- Beet Greens (Cooked)

- Arugula (Rocket)

- Brussels Sprouts (Cooked)

# Chapter 8 - Sleep Your Way To Weight Loss

Getting enough sleep is crucial to losing weight.

When you don't get enough sleep, your body is stressed out and releases a hormone called cortisol. This hormone leads to weight gain indirectly.

What most people fail to realize is that being constantly deprived of sleep will take a toll on your health in the long run.

Research has shown that people who have less sleep eat more, feel hungrier and generally consume 350 calories more than required. Those who stay awake late often find themselves consuming snacks and heavy meals often.

Your body's insulin sensitivity and glucose tolerance levels will drop. This is bad since your body will go into fat storage mode instead of being in fat burning mode. When your insulin sensitivity is down, you will store fat much more easily. The same applies for glucose tolerance.

Lack of sleep also increases the body's stress hormone, cortisol. Once again the body's fat burning ability decreases or in a worst case scenario, just completely stops.

If you're eating on a caloric deficit and training daily, your body is already stressed out. It needs sleep to rest and repair itself. Not to mention de-stress.

There is a reason it is referred to as "beauty sleep".

All the best attempts at losing weight will be hampered if you can't afford to get enough sleep at night. Power naps during the day will not cut it.

You need sleep at night for at least 7 hours. Most people claim to get by on less. They may... but at a price to their health in the long run.

Aim to be more productive so that you get more work done in the office and don't have to stay late. Stop watching late night TV and do not work out too close to bedtime. Ideally, you should be working out in the day.

Try and meditate to free your mind from the daily stresses of life. Remember, even if you win the rat race, you're still a rat. There is more to life than deadlines, targets and appraisals.

Get enough sleep and you will find it much easier to shed the fat. The power of a good night's sleep should never be underestimated.

Do ensure that you're getting at least 6 to 8 hours of sleep daily. Don't burn the candle at both ends when you're on a weight loss journey.

# Chapter 9 - Finding the Time

Most women are hard-pressed for time. You could be the mother of a newly born child who needs your full attention. Or you might be a career woman with demanding deadlines and you still need to juggle your duties as a wife.

We live in a fast paced world. Everybody is running the rat race to be the best rat. Time is a precious commodity that never seems to be enough. So what do you do?

You improvise. That's what you do.

To put things in perspective, you must realize that there are 24 hours in a day. A one hour workout is 4 percent of your day. A 15 minute workout is one percent of your day. An eight minute workout is "half a percent" of your day!

But what can I achieve in 8 minutes? A lot!

Anybody no matter how busy, can squeeze in 8 minutes. 8 minutes is too much? How about 4 minutes? What?! 4 Minutes?

Yes. 4 minutes of Tabata protocol. You can Google it to find out more. The point here is that you can cause a metabolic boost to your body and put it in fat burning mode within 4 minutes and you will be in a fat burning state for hours. Will it be easy? No. But it will be effective.

If you do not have time for one hour long workouts, do quick bursts of 15 minutes or even less. The difference is that the shorter workouts will have to be more intense. However, it will be for a short while only.

There are also other methods to ensure that you burn more calories. Get yourself a pair of ankle weights and wear them throughout the day.

You will burn more calories when you walk and move. If you're a stay at home mom, get a haversack and add some weight in it. Throw in a telephone directory or 2 and wear the haversack.

The added weight will make everything more difficult and you will be burning more calories because of the added resistance.

Get yourself a Fitbit which will track the number of steps you take daily. Aim to increase the number of steps by 100 everyday. Climb the stairs instead of using the elevator. Walk to the supermarket if you can.

If you're the mother of a newborn, get an infant sling and place your baby in it. Then proceed for a 30 minute walk. Excellent exercise for you and the baby gets a breath of fresh air too.

You may not have enough time. Yet, with a bit of imagination, you can incorporate many little practices and changes in your life to burn more calories. Once you have that done, get a journal and record your hourly activities.

See where your time goes. "Oh look! I'm watching Sex and the City reruns daily!"... ah hah! A time waster right there. Cut it out and spend that 30 minutes exercising. It will do you more good than watching, Samantha, trying to get it on with all the guys in New York.

Do whatever you can with whatever time you have. Even if it's only 4 minutes.

# Chapter 10 - Structuring Your Workouts

The importance of following a good training regimen that not only boosts your stamina, but also strengthens and tones your body cannot be over emphasized.

Cardio is a great way to burn calories and lose weight.

Millions of women around the world focus ONLY on cardio workouts. This is a mistake because strength training is crucial for weight loss too.

The more lean muscle mass your body has, the more calories it burns while at rest.

That essentially means you'll be a fat burning machine throughout the day.

The best way to structure your workout will be to have 3 cardio sessions a week and two resistance training sessions.

## The Power of Fasted Cardio

Cardio is extremely effective when done on an empty stomach.

You may have heard that exercising on an empty stomach is great for weight loss. However, the idea of a strenuous workout so soon after waking doesn't appeal to most people.

The good news is that it does NOT have to be strenuous.

In fact, it's best to keep things relatively light.

One of the best ways of losing weight is to go for a brisk walk first thing in the morning. A short 20 to 30 minute walk is ideal.

You should be able to hold a conversation while walking. You shouldn't be exerting yourself to a point where you're panting and gasping.

We're not aiming for high intensity here.

When you wake up in the morning, your body is in a fasted state. Your glycogen levels are low and the food in your body would have been digested.

This means that your body will be forced to burn fat for fuel while you walk. So, during the 20 to 30 minutes that you're walking, your body is burning its fat stores for fuel.

This is a very powerful method and since it's not strenuous, you can do it daily.

The morning walk will also boost your metabolic rate and you'll burn more calories throughout the day.

If you don't wish to walk, you may swim or use a stationary bike. As long as it's a cardio activity that's at a moderate pace, your body will burn fat and your efforts will pay off.

You may wish to engage in strength training or a short high intensity interval training later in the day. That's perfectly fine because the morning workout is just meant to speed up the fat burning process.

It's an additional technique to help you reach your weight goals faster. This is such an easy method that anyone can do it.

If all you can manage is a 10-minute walk, then just do 10 minutes. With time, you can slowly progress to 20 or 30 minutes. There's really no need to go above 30 minutes.

Give this method a try and within a couple of weeks, you will see the difference.

## Weight training

Many women worry about getting bulky and muscular like men if they were to train with weights. This assumption is false.

Even men struggle with gaining muscle. Women who train with weights will look leaner and more defined but they will not become manly.

You can cast aside all worries about looking like a female bodybuilder.

Bodyweight training such as squats, push-ups, lunges, dips and pull ups are great ways to work your muscles and joints.

It's crucial to work your muscles or they will atrophy with age. Look for exercises that tone your thighs, butt and arms.

These are common problem areas for many women. While cardio will help you shed the fat, strength training will give you the curves and definition that will make you look fit, healthy and radiant.

A short 10 to 15 minute full body workout done early in the day will work miracles. This type of workout is known as HIIT… High Intensity Interval Training.

Here's the kicker. You can even do a HIIT workout in one spot and still sweat like crazy.

For example, let's look at this workout circuit.

Sit Ups – 45 seconds

Burpees – 45 seconds

Jump Squats – 45 seconds

Push Ups – 45 seconds

High Knees – 45 seconds

Jumping Jacks – 45 seconds

Burpees – 45 seconds

Alternating Lung Jumps – 45 seconds

Sit ups – 45 seconds

Push Ups – 45 seconds

Each exercise will have 15 seconds of rest before you move on to the next. You could do this workout in a cubicle. It takes up that little space... BUT... most people will not be able to even make it to the 9th exercise.

Why?

Because of the intensity. You need to go as hard as you can go. There is no taking it easy. If all you have is 10 minutes, then it MUST be a hard 10 minutes.

The good news is that this is just 10 minutes. You'll be in the 'hurt box' during this time but you need to keep telling yourself... "It's only 10 minutes! I can do this."

You could complete a workout within a commercial break. It's that fast. If you do this workout early in the day, your body will be in fat burning mode throughout the day because of the intensity.

It creates a situation in your body known as post-exercise oxygen consumption. That means your body will be burning calories at an accelerated rate for 10 to even 14 hours after your workout is over.

It's amazing what just 10 minutes can do.

The reason you do it early in the day is because your metabolism drops the moment you go to bed. By completing your training early in the day, you'll reap maximum rewards.

It's also worth noting that it's best that you make these short workouts full body workouts. Do compound movements such as squats, jumps push ups, etc.

By recruiting as many muscles in your body as you can, you'll be ensuring that your workout is engaging the whole body.

Don't just try to wing it with simple exercises such as dumbbell curls and call it a day. All you have is 10 minutes. You have to make it count.

Even 3 of these short workouts a week will transform your body within a month. Go ahead and give them a try. You will be amazed.

Do remember to have 2 rest days a week. You can split them up or you can have both days back to back. It's really up to you.

What matters is that you take a break every week so that your muscles and central nervous system have time to recover. By going too hard without rest, your body will get tired and stressed out.

You may end up hitting a weight loss plateau and once that happens, you won't lose weight no matter what you do.

You will then need to take a 4 to 5 day break just to recover. This will slow down your progress and you may even gain weight.

Take a 2 day break every week.

Do your research online and find the best resistance training and cardio workouts.

Vary your workouts and challenge your body. You'll get stronger and leaner in no time at all.

# Chapter 11 - Putting the Fun In It

Make your exercise sessions fun. Find a workout buddy if you need one.

Don't do the same workouts daily. Monotony can discourage even the most enthusiastic woman.

Try something new. Maybe yoga at the gym... or kickboxing.

You could try rock-climbing too!

Feel like dancing? Check out Shaun T's workouts and follow along.

The key here is to keep moving. Your caloric deficit will cause weight loss no matter what you do.

The exercise is just to speed up the process.

Do whatever you like. Cycling, running, swimming.

What matters is that you MOVE daily. A sedentary lifestyle is what causes obesity.

Keep moving and keep it fun.

# Chapter 12 - Dealing with Slip Ups

It's going to happen. Sooner or later it definitely is going to happen. "What's going to happen?" you ask.

You're going to slip-up on your diet and eat something you know you shouldn't or you may not do a workout that you know you should.

It happens to almost all of us. How you proceed from a slip-up makes all the difference to whether you succeed in your weight loss journey or fail miserably.

Let's look at slipping up with your diet first. When you go on a weight loss journey, it usually involves eating less than you're accustomed to, in order to create a caloric deficit. You'll also need to focus on eating foods that are healthy and wholesome while avoiding processed and junk food.

However, the body is already used to eating without much thought and you're probably addicted to processed and junk food without even realizing it. Millions of people are, and when they try to ditch these unhealthy foods, they get cravings and mood swings.

The key point is to make the changes gradual. Only aim for a 500 calorie deficit daily. This is a manageable amount and you will not be feeling pangs of hunger.

You may feel a little peckish but it will be manageable. If you cut your calories too drastically, you will be feeling hungry all the time and this is sheer mental and physical torture.

Changing your foods overnight causes the same problem. Your body is not used to it. Aim to gradually reduce consumption of the bad foods and replace them with good ones.

If you drink 3 cans of soda daily, cut it down to 2 for a week and then bring it down to 1 can... and finally, put an end to the soda habit. Don't just give up sodas overnight.

Problems arise when people try to do too much too soon. They make things so challenging that compliance becomes a nightmare. People aim for perfection.

Sooner or later they lose the battle of wills within themselves and give in to temptation and eat a greasy cheeseburger and fries or they polish off an entire bag of cookies.

When that happens, they feel guilty and think that they have failed. They then believe that they're destined to be fat and they throw in the towel and give up on their goal. This happens to millions of people and is the reason why so many people quit.

The first point to note when you slip-up is that you made a single mistake. You have not failed yet. You only fail when you give up. If you accidentally dropped your mobile phone, wouldn't you quickly pick it up, dust it off and keep it safely?

Surely you wouldn't keep dropping it and smashing it because of the first accident.

In the same way, acknowledge your slip-up and move on. Tell yourself that you will be more mindful of what you eat. Ease up on your stringent diet and allow flexibility while maintaining a caloric deficit. Do not deprive yourself of too much too soon.

As for your workouts, the same mindset should apply. If you miss a workout today, make sure you do one the next day. Never ever miss more than 3 workout sessions in a row or you'll conveniently fall off track and it will be very tough to go back.

If you dread exercising, you're either pushing yourself too hard or you're engaged in an activity that you have no interest in.

Exercise is meant to boost your metabolic rate and increase fat burning. Your diet and caloric deficit is what really matters when it comes to fat loss.

Missed workouts and diet mistakes are not the end of the world and should definitely not be the end of your weight loss journey.

It is a journey and it's inevitable that you get lost along the way every now and then. If you stay on track and keep going despite your setbacks, you will reach your goal. That's almost always how most people reach their goals. Keep your chin up and keep moving forward.

# Chapter 13 - Taking Time to Smell the Roses

There will be times when you just feel like giving up. This is normal.

What you need to do is relax and enjoy the process. Be satisfied with even a pound of weight loss. You can lose more the following week.

What matters is that you know that you'll get there and you must stay positive.

Don't obsess over your weight. Maintain the caloric deficit, do your workouts, drink enough water, get enough sleep, make your workouts fun... and relax.

You will reach your goal. Watch a movie or a comedy to de-stress. Go on a vacation but don't throw your diet away.

Always keep your chin up and keep going forward. Visualize where you want to be... and you'll get there.

# Chapter 14 - Getting There and Staying There

Most women who lose weight often gain it back after a while. Even people on TV shows such as The Biggest Loser gained all the fat they all once the show ended.

In order to stay slim, you need to change your lifestyle.

You'll need to practice whatever you're learned in this book for life.

Once you reach your ideal weight, you will need to consume your calories at maintenance level. This will ensure that you neither gain nor lose more weight.

Keep doing the workouts you're doing to stay fit.

You'll always have to be on the ball. A rolling stone gathers no moss... so you'll need to keep at it.

It took you so much effort to get to your weight loss goals... don't lose it all by going back to your old ways.

Eat healthy, stay active... and be happy.

www.ingramcontent.com/pod-product-compliance
Lightning Source LLC
Chambersburg PA
CBHW080629030426
42336CB00018B/3132